NATURAL ESSENTIAL OILS AND AROMATHERAPY

FOR BEGINNERS

Disclaimer

This e-book is the property of the author. Any publication, in part or as a whole, needs to be first properly authorized. This includes digital and mechanical reproduction. The author has made all possible efforts to provide accurate information, however, any changes in the future are unforeseeable and thus subject to change.

This e-book is for educational purposes only and should be taken as such. Do not substitute the contents of this e-book for professional or medical advice. The author will not be responsible for any damage incurred due to the misappropriation of any of the contents of this e-book.

What You Will Find Inside

Natural Essential Oils and Aromatherapy for Beginners is a basic guide to the history, purpose and benefits of essential oils and aromatherapy as a whole. Aromatherapy is being used today for relieving physical, psychological and emotional stress.

Essential oils are extracted from flowers, bark, roots and stems of various plants. This e-book is your first step towards the understanding of these oils and how to optimally use them to better the quality of your life. This book is both informative and educational and provides a step by step guide to aromatherapy. It includes:

1. Introduction to aromatherapy and essential oils

2. Purpose and history of aromatherapy

3. Benefits of essential oils

4. Properties of various essential oils

5. Methods of making essential oils

6. Guide on how to properly apply and use various essential oils

Table of Contents

Chapter 1 - Introduction to

Aromatherapy

Have you ever wondered why nature has become all so beautiful again? Why is it that people opt for those natural wonders that are secluded and untouched by human technology when planning holidays? Many even opt out of taking their basic 'necessities' like mobile phones and laptops with them. Why is it that nature is so desirable again?

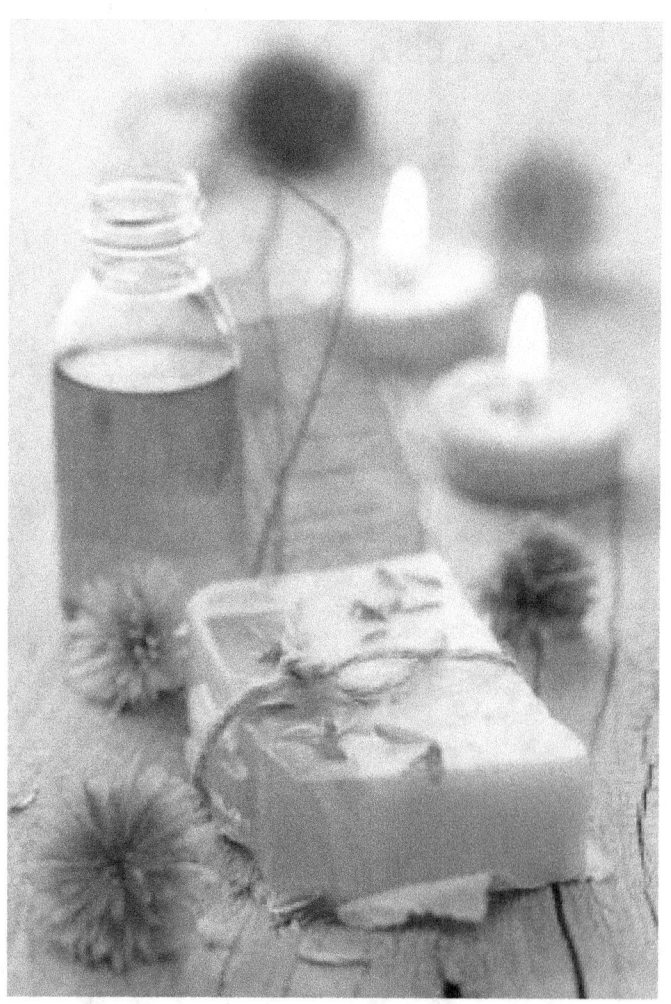

Many claim that technology has evolved much too quickly when compared to the human body and psychology. Our bodies, which have been programmed to behave in certain manners and respond to specific medications are unable to achieve the same results with the synthetic alternatives being offered today.

Hence, the 'organic' life or Paleolithic lifestyle choices are often opted for as an escape routein order to get back in touch with what feels natural to our bodies.

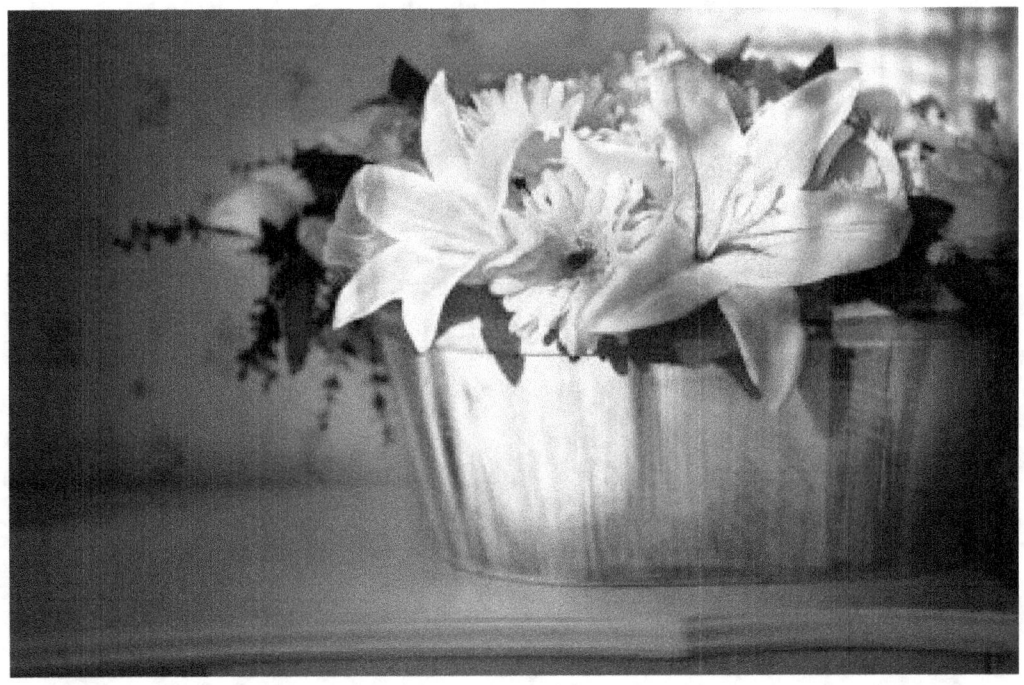

Aromatherapy is not a new phenomenon. It has been in use since the ancient times when tree gums, wood and fragrant leaves were burned for aroma during the Neolithic times. However, it took a hiatus during the early 20th century when the mass production of medicines became popular due to industrialization.

In recent times, however, it has had a major comeback and has again been identified as an effective, organic and natural remedy for infections, stress and overall cognitive functioning.

What are Essential Oils?

Aromatherapy uses essential oils of various plants to offer relief. Essential oils are extracted from flowers, wood, leaves, trees and specific plants to form a highly concentrated oil. There are various methods for extracting essential oils at smaller as well as larger scales. The primary reason essential oils have become widely popular is because they tend to offer no side effects while providing long term relief.

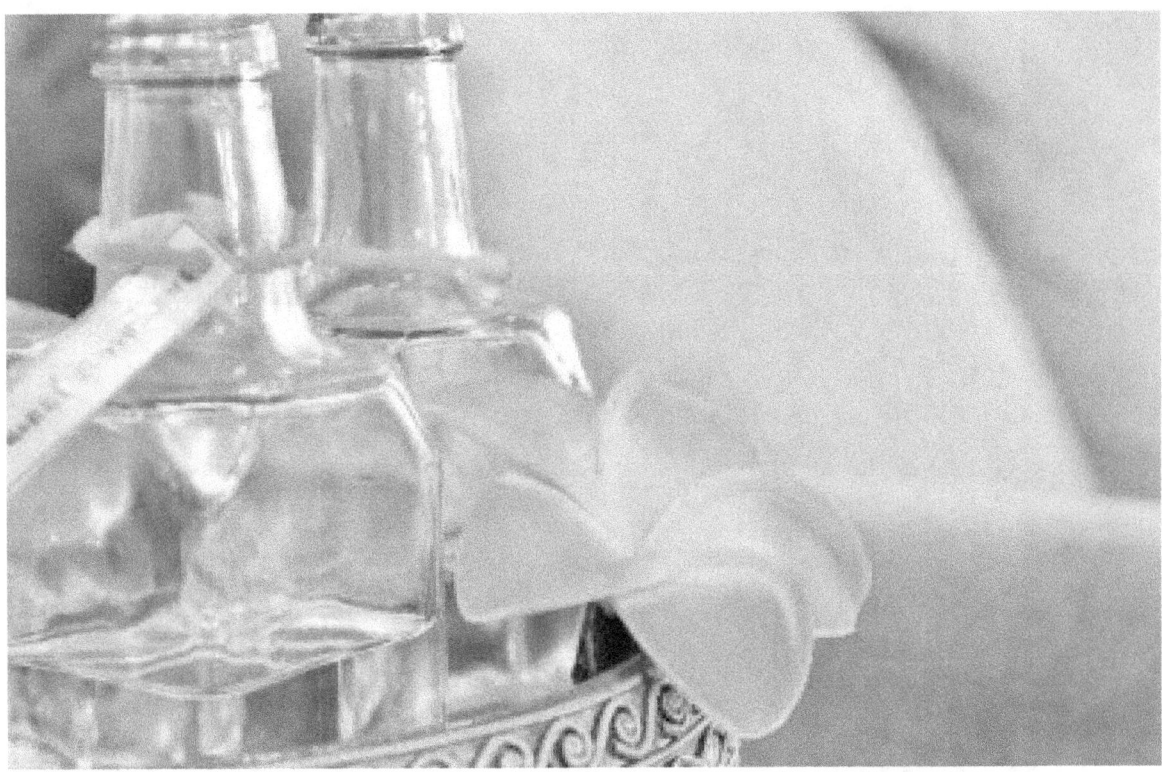

An essential oil can typically contain more than a hundred different chemical compounds. Each compound proposes certain characteristics and properties that are beneficial for both body and mind. Almost every essential oil contains antiviral, antiseptic and antibacterial properties.

Essential oils provide a more holistic approach to treating various ailments using natural ingredients. So if you are looking for a natural and organic way of treating basic ailments like depression, stress, anxiety, chronic pain, infections, burns, etc. then aromatherapy is the most effective and safe option out there.

History of Aromatherapy

Like most new inventions from ancient times, aromatherapy too was discovered by accidently figuring out that specific woods gave away a sweet aromatic fragrance when burnt. The word perfume itself is derived from the Latin phrase 'per fumum' which means 'through smoke'.

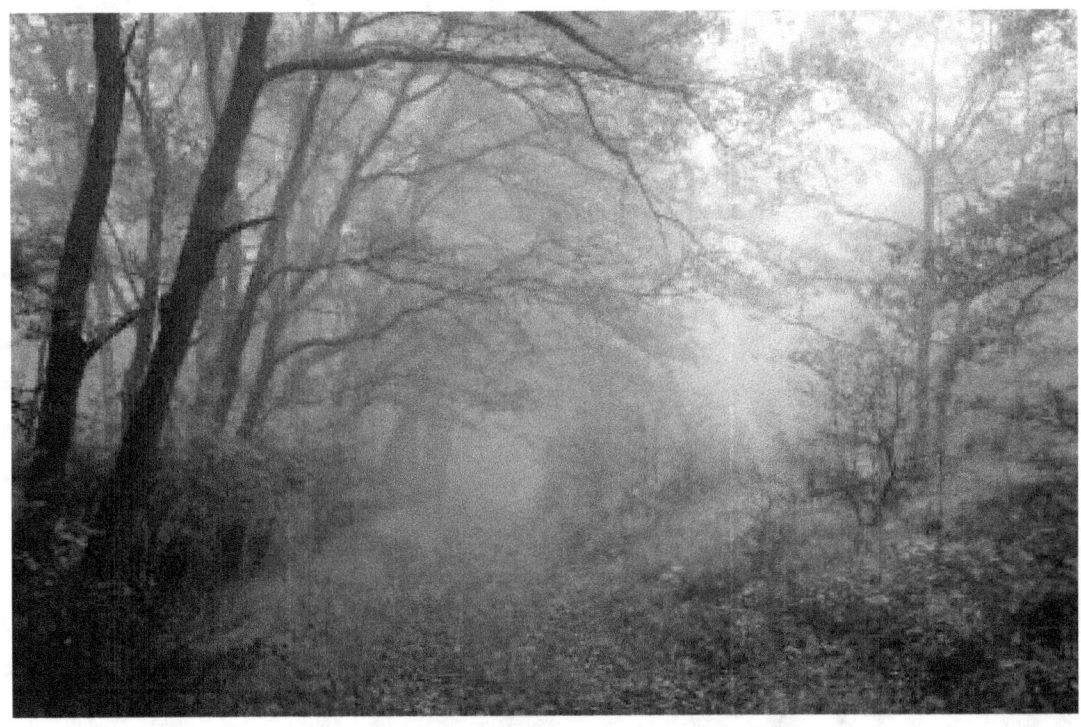

As far back as 4000 B.C.E., Neolithic tribes heated particular plants, leaves and flowers with animal fat for healing specific ailments. History of aromatherapy can easily be dated back to those times. However, the more documented history of aromatherapy is dated back to 2,000 years ago by the Egyptians. They used balsamic materials for their religious rituals. Resins like myrrh and frankincense were blended with oils and spices to be burnt during ceremonies for heightened spiritual consciousness.

The father of modern medicine, Hippocrates also encouraged people to have scented baths and daily massages to lead a healthier lifestyle. He claimed that burning plants on street corners could prevent plague from spreading.

Avicenna in the 11th Century invented the steam distillation method that greatly helped in extracting essential oils from plants. The first lavender oil was made in the 12th century using the same method by Hildegard of Bingen.

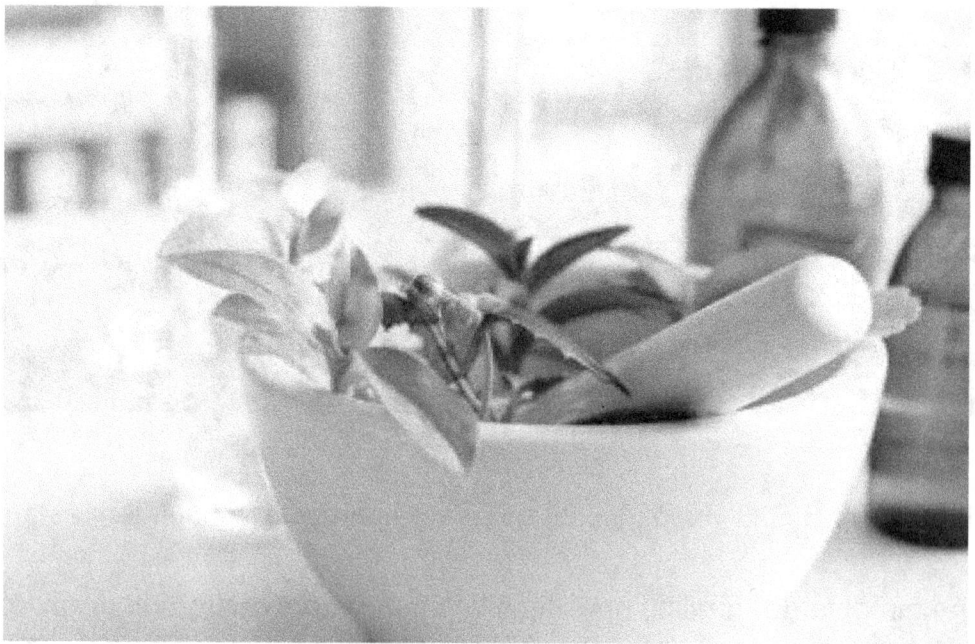

Herbalists Gerard, Culpeper and Parkinson extensively wrote about the use of medicinal plants in the 16th century. Essential oils since then became highly popular and were widely used for aromatic, treatment and relaxation purposes until the 20th century, when chemistry made way to more synthetic elements for curing diseases.

However, soon people realized that these elements not only cause side effects, but can also be harmful. These medicines too are evolving into using more natural elements to lessen the side effects and be closer to nature to be more effective.

R.M. Gattefosse, a French Chemist, is responsible for establishing aromatherapy as we know it today. He had burned his hand while working in his laboratory one day and had plunged his hand into the lavender oil container placed nearby.

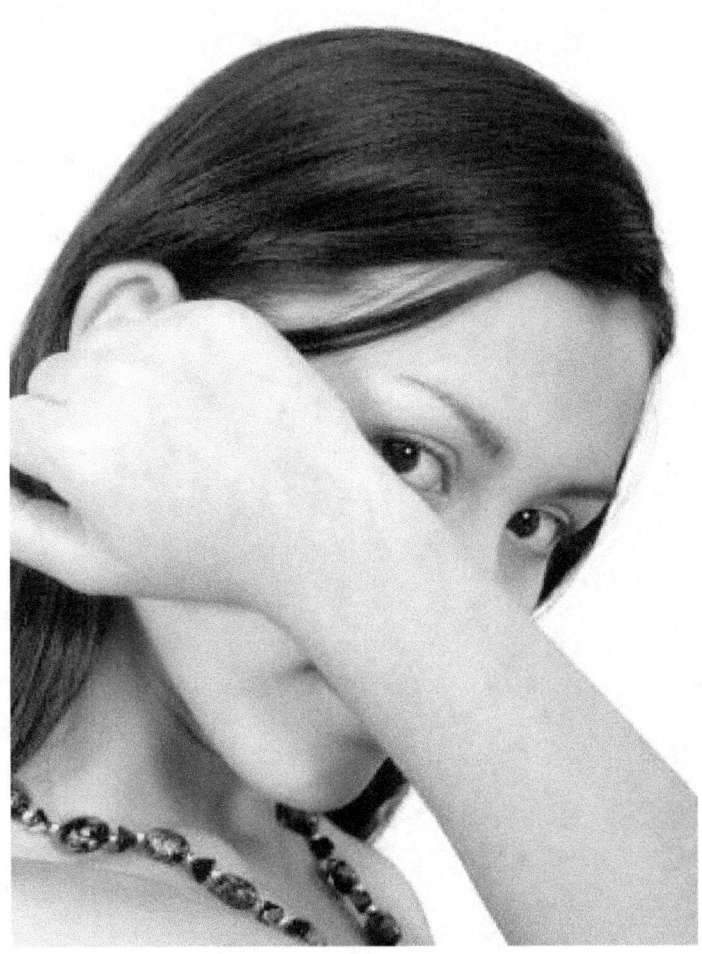

The oil was highly effective in not only relieving the pain, but speeding up the healing process. He then decided to switch his study to natural oils, or what he termed as 'aromatherapy.'

Soon the phenomenon was caught on by other scientists and biochemists and thus the interest in essential oils regained its status as one of the most naturally effective forms available for healing of the mind and body.

Advantages of Aromatherapy

Aromatherapy is a vast generalization for all the beneficial properties of various essential oils. They can be used to clean the house, improve memory, relieve discomfort, stimulate cancer patients and lift spirits. And this is just an overview.

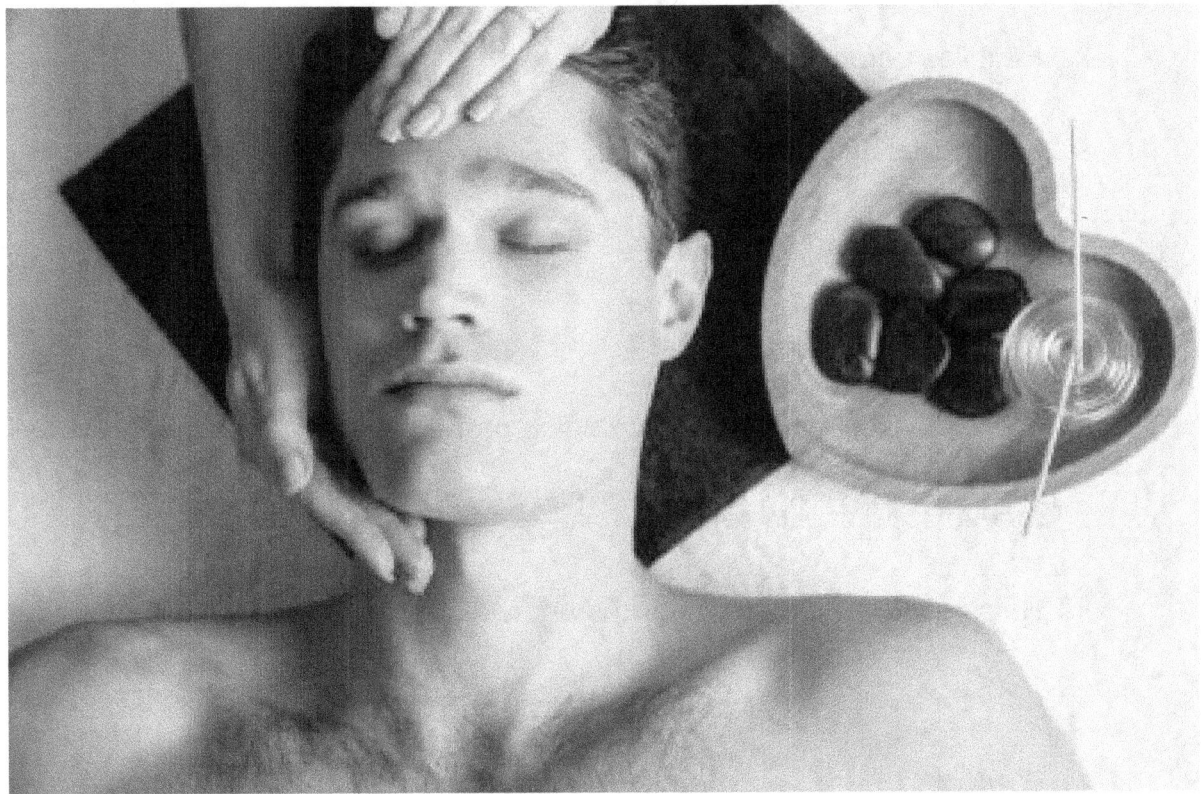

Aromatherapy is highly advantageous for your skin, hair, mood and even relationships. Following are some of the many benefits of using essential oils in your daily life:

1. You can use it to sanitize your house.

2. Strengthens immune system.

3. It eliminates fungal infections, bacteria and viruses.

4. Relaxes muscles, heightens the feeling of well being and enhances mood.

5. It induces sleep.

6. It relieves chronic pain.

7. It does not have any side effects.

8. Relieves chronic pain.

9. It improves digestive system functioning.

10. Strengthens the respiratory system.

11. Safe for children and pets.

12. Prevents wrinkles and has anti aging properties like promoting regeneration of skin cells.

13. Helps soothe and cleanse burns and wounds.

14. Penetrates and repairs damaged tissue.

Chapter 2 - Aromatherapy Basics

How are Essential Oils Produced?

Essential oils are produced by extracting highly concentrated oils from aromatic plants. There are more than 700 different known plants that can be used to extract effective essential oils.

There are plenty of ways to extract essential oils, however the most popular method remains distillation. Distillation converts the liquid from the plant or other source into a vapor. The vapor is then condensed back into liquid form. It is the most cost effective method of extraction for essential oils available.

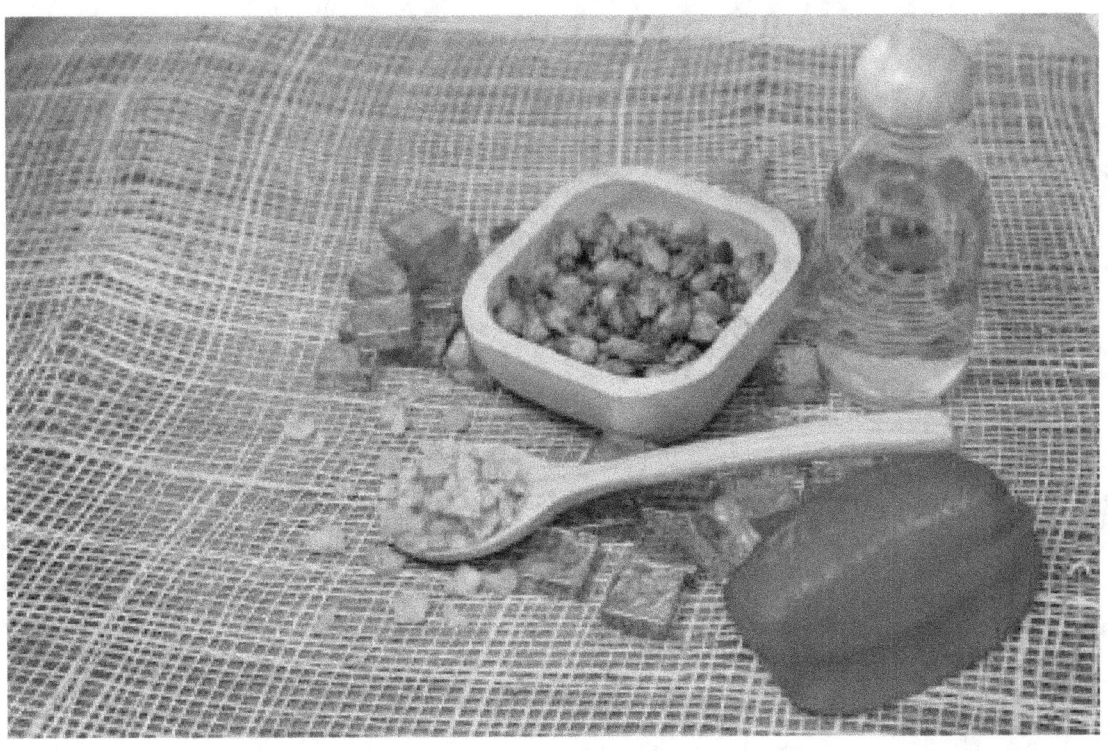

There are a number of different forms of distillation also including water distillation, steam distillation, fractional distillation, hydro diffusion, rectification, water and steam combined distillation and cohobation. The method used primarily depends on the wood, flower or plant that is being processed.

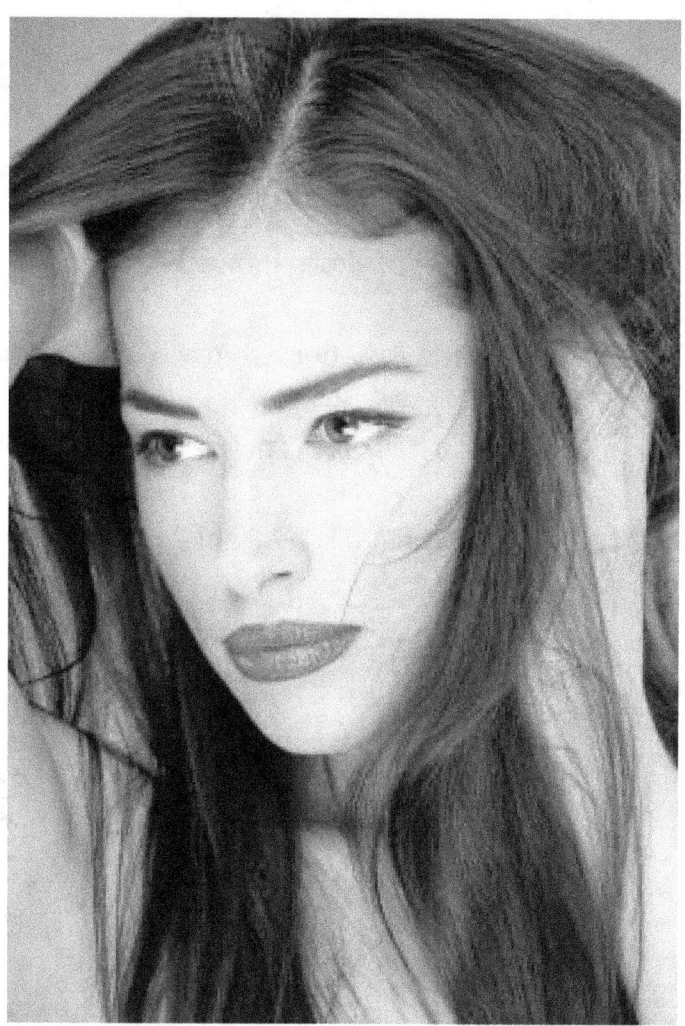

There are other methods available for extraction too including, expressions and solvent extractions. Expression is a cold pressed method that is generally used for extracting essential oils from citrus fruits. There are three different methods for extracting using expression. These include: machine abrasion, sponge expression and Ecuelle a piquer.

Solvent extractions are used for the extraction of essential oils from botanical materials. There are four different methods employed for solvent extraction including: maceration, solvent, enfleurage and Hypercritical carbon dioxide CO_2.

How Do they Work?

Essential oils are miniscule in molecular size which makes them easy to be absorbed. The skin absorbs the oil, which then penetrates into the blood stream and eliminates waste material and rejuvenates the skin.

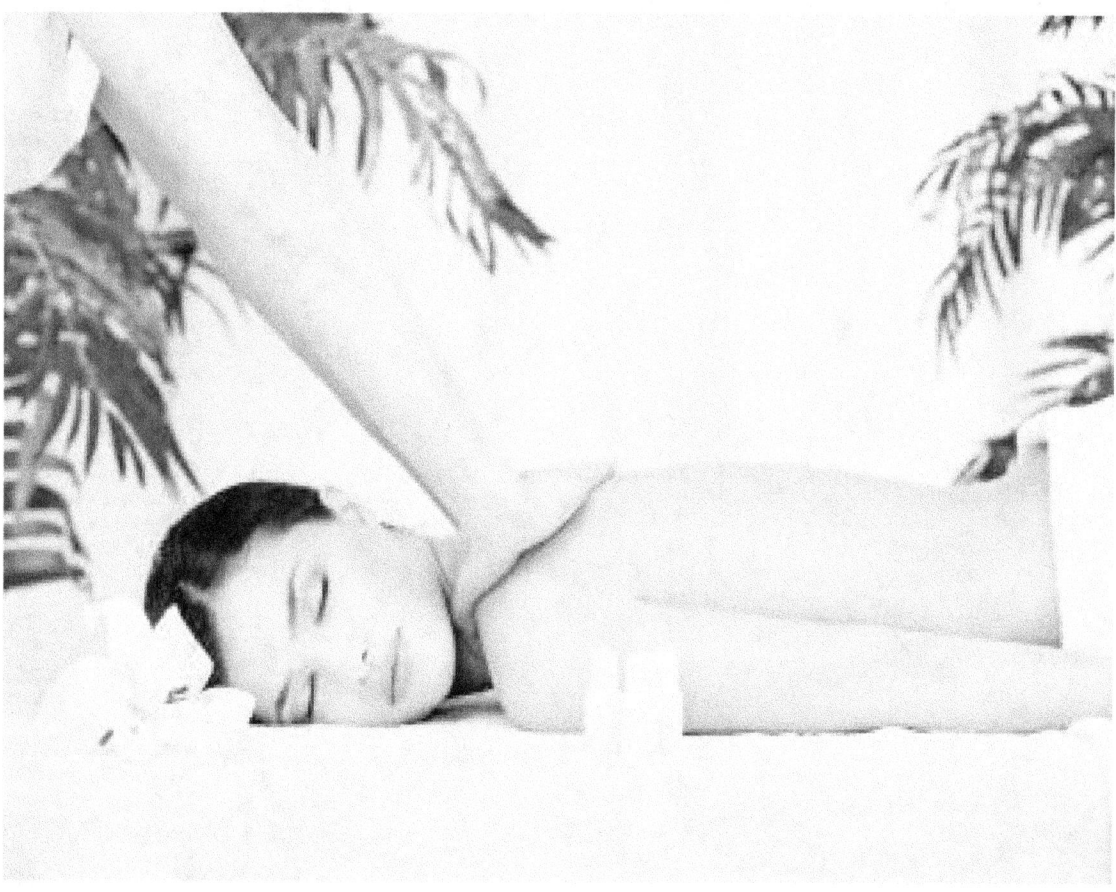

A standard 30-40 minute massage using essential oil can be beneficial for mental clarity, de-stressing and overall health and well being of the human mind, body and spirit. It is therefore no surprise that essential oils have become the go-to solution for individuals leading hectic and busy lifestyles.

Essential oils are usually mixed with **carrier oils** before applying. Essential oils on their own can be quite strong, thus carrier oils like almond oil or olive oil are used to dilute the essential oil before application. Some carrier oils work better when paired with specific essential oils and even assist in relieving pain and stress. Make sure you understand the characteristics of both the carrier oil and the essential oil before mixing them.

Chapter 3 – Applications

Essential oils are used in a number of different ways. Although, the most common usage is through body massages, it is not the only method of application. Following are a number of different ways you can use essential oils in your daily life:

Bath

Simply add a few droplets of your desired essential oil into a bath tub filled with warm water and soak yourself in it. Only a few droplets of essential oil will greatly assist in relieving stress by relaxing your body and inducing your brain. If you aren't up for a long cozy bath, you can achieve the same effects by using a towel and a bowl of warm water.

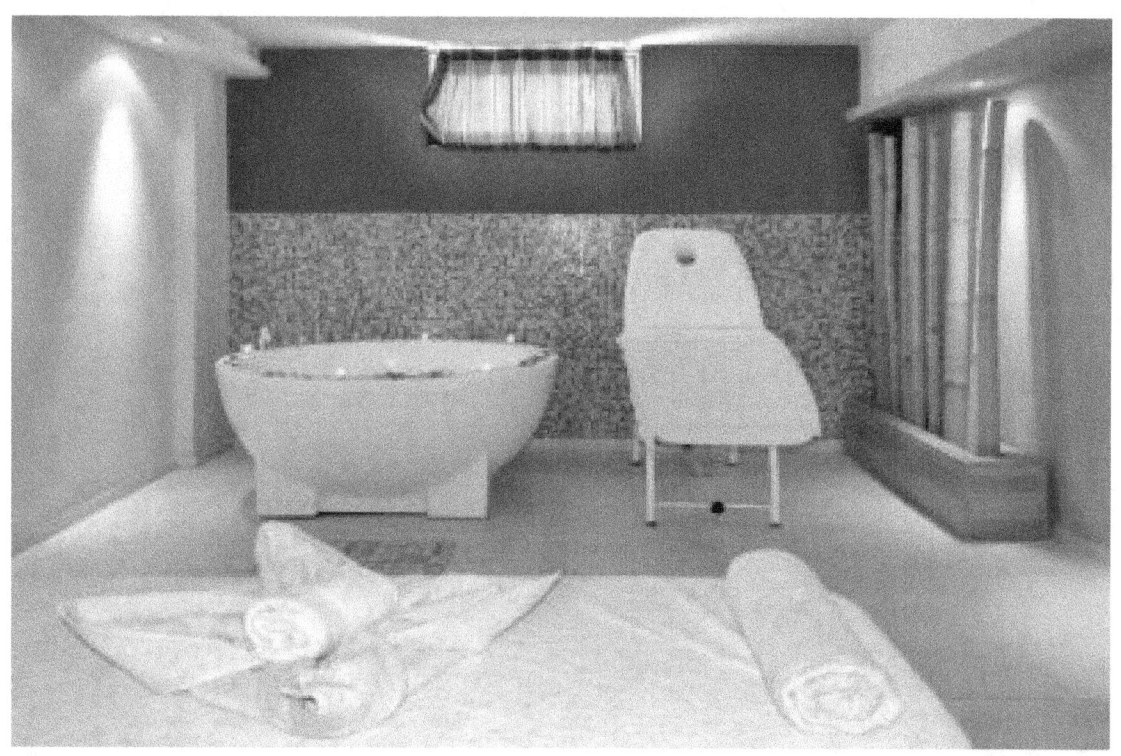

Just add a few droplets of your choice of essential oil in a bowl of warm water. Take

a cloth or towel and swish it across the bowl of water and apply it to your neck, back,

arms, legs, abdomen, etc. If you are experiencing pain, you can apply the wet cloth

to the desired area to ease the pain.

Body

Essential oils are applied in various forms to the body for a number of different reasons. You can use it as a facial steam, hair oil or massage your body with it. Add the carrier oil of your choice to the essential oil and massage it in the desired area.

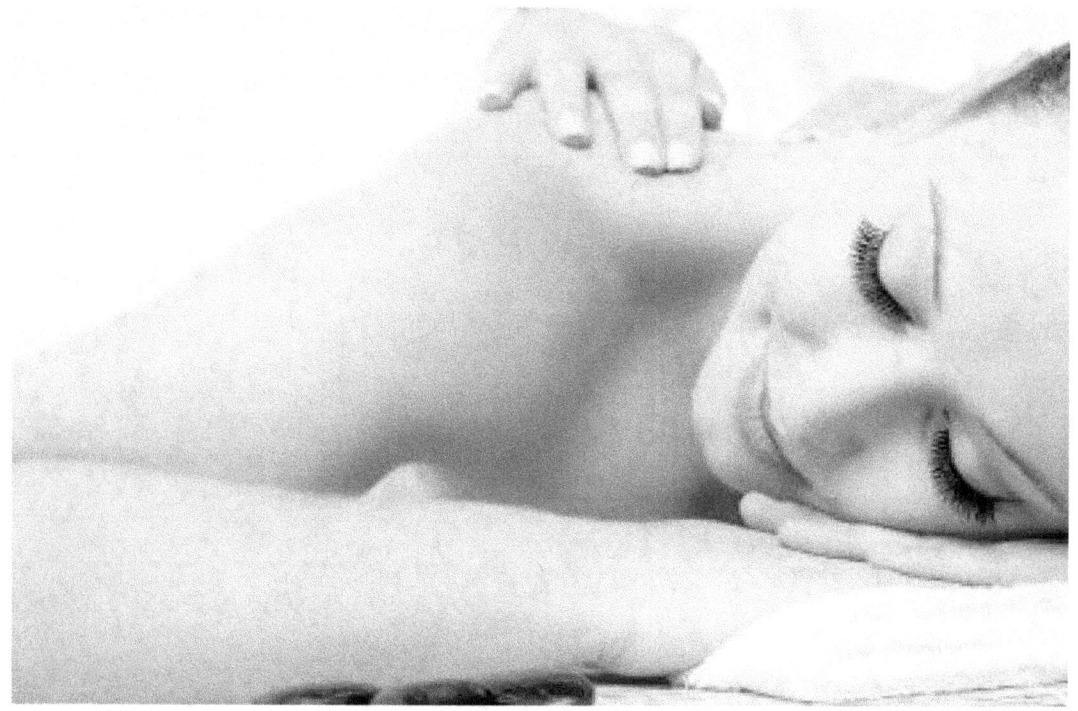

1. For skin care, mix essential oil into a carrier oil, lotion or cream and massage it on your face and body.

2. You can also make a facial masque by adding a few droplets of the essential oil in egg whites or clay.

3. Add a few droplets of essential oil in boiling water and take a facial steam to rejuvenate your skin.

4. Add two to three drops of essential oil to the bristle of a bath brush and brush it over your skin. This method is called **dry brushing** and is highly popular for relaxing the muscles. Make sure you brush lightly. Ideally, you should start from your toes towards your heart, then from the tips of your fingers towards your heart. Do not dry brush your face or neck.

Diffusers and Candles

Candles and diffusers using essential oils are highly popular. Don't mistake these for scented candles. Although essential oil candles and diffusers are scented, candles can be scented using other, non-effective methods also. Diffusers and candles give out a pleasant scent and have great calming properties that are highly effective in relieving stress.

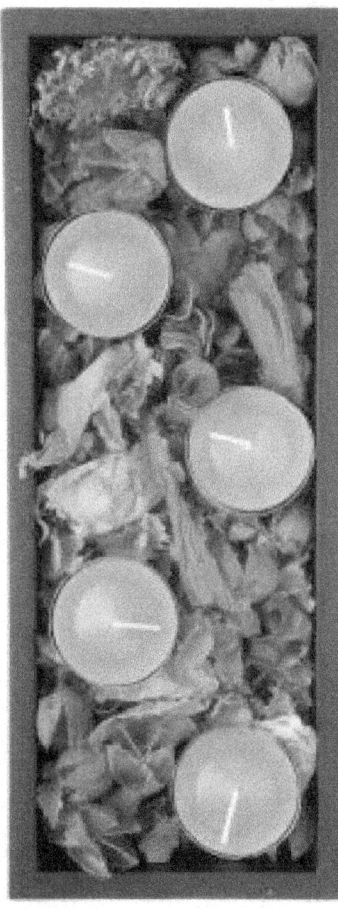 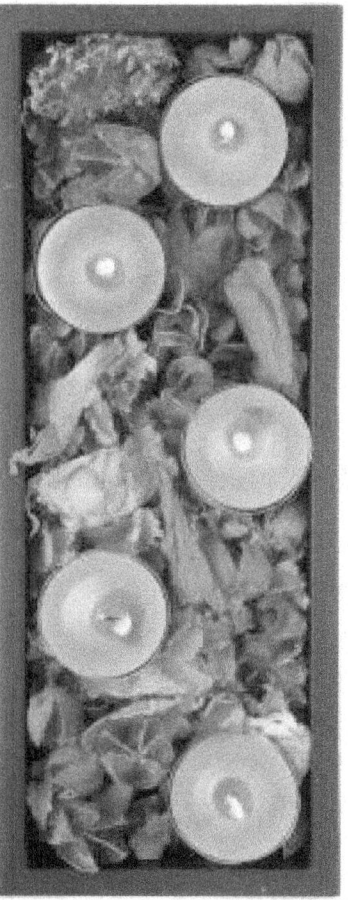

Nebulizing Diffusers

Nebulizing diffusers are devices that are used to treat bronchial problems and sinus.

Simply add a few droplets of essential oil into your device and use it according to the

manufacturer's instructions.

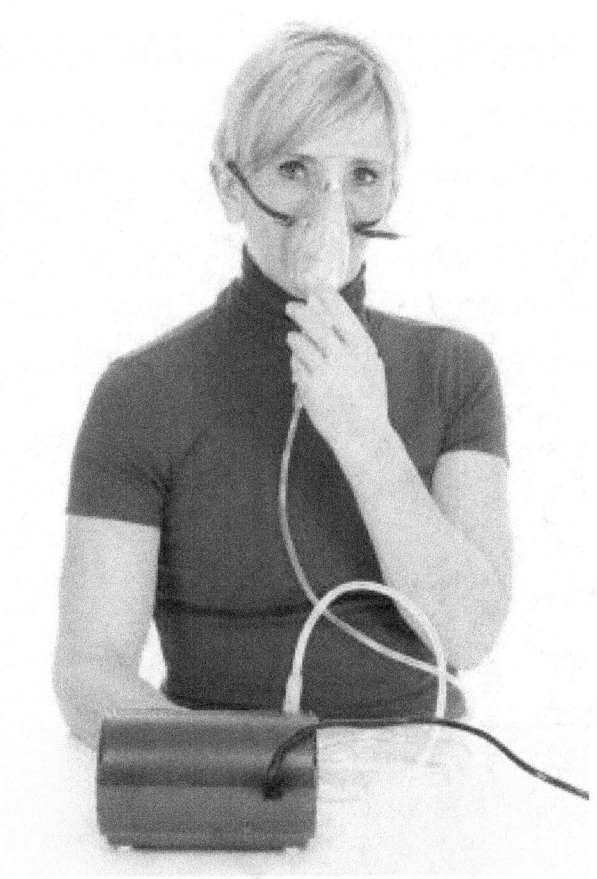

Not all essential oils are effective or even recommended to be used with nebulizers,

so make sure you fully understand the properties of the essential oil of your choice

and your condition before using them.

Household Items

Essential oils are used in laundry, cleaning the house and even for washing dishes.

Most essential oils antibacterial properties makes them effective for disinfecting the

house and clothing. And the lingering aromatic smell is an added bonus.

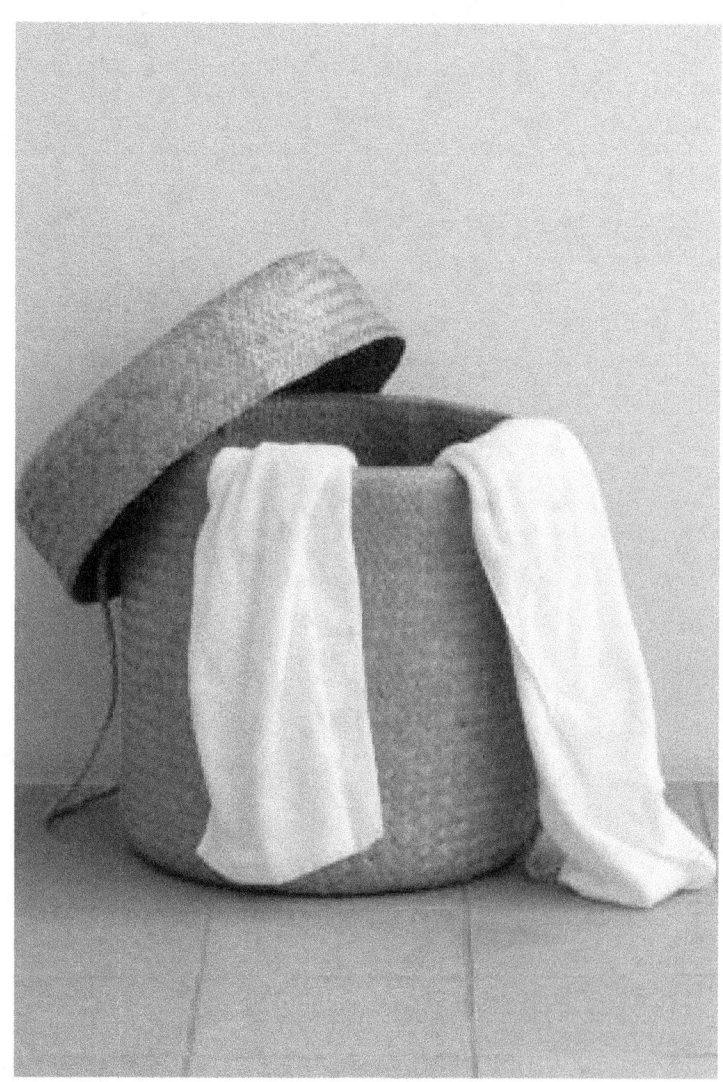

Chapter 4 – Properties of Some Popular Essential Oils

Primarily, the effectiveness of the essential oil will depend on the quality of the product. Scented products like oil and soaps do not necessarily mean that they are essential oils. Sometimes, manufacturers use flavoring or perfumery to enhance the scent of the oil and categorize them as 'essential oils'. However, essential oils are only undiluted extracts that have not been tampered with.

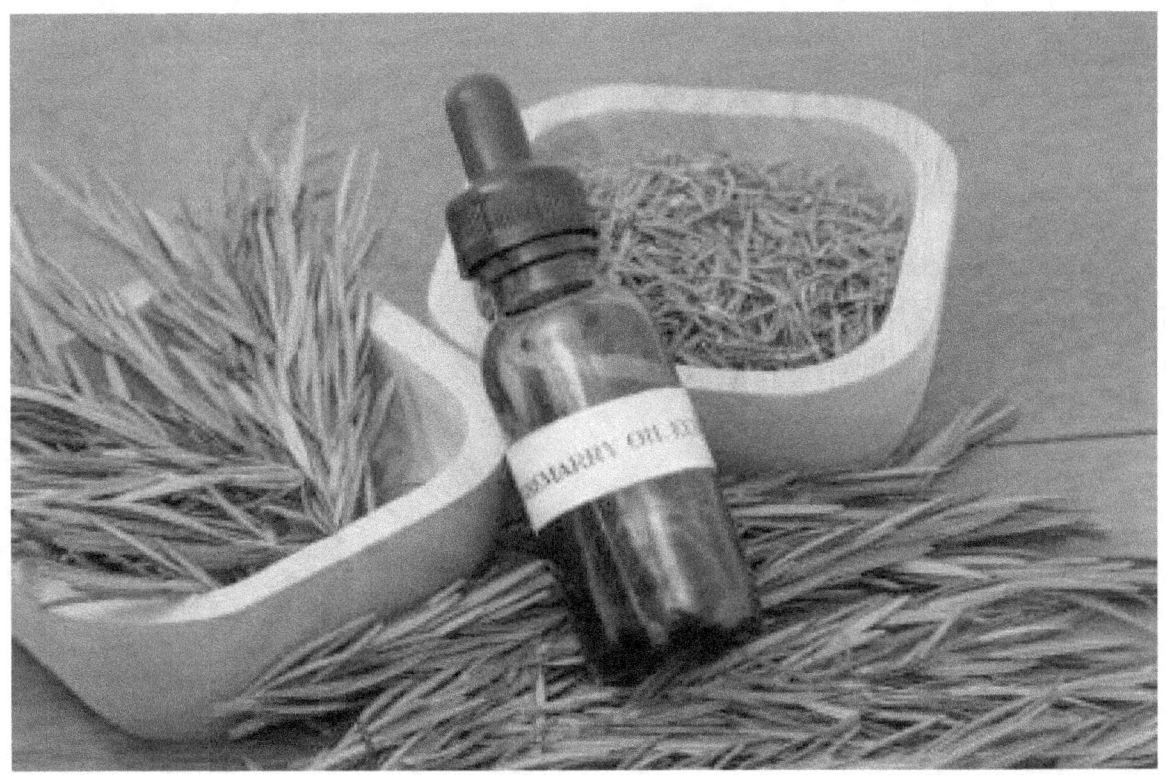

Make sure you read the label before purchasing an essential oil, because those that have been treated aren't as effective as pure essential oils. Or you can extract the essential oils yourself using the extraction kits available in the market.

Essential oils serve different purposes; while some are great for relaxation, others have effective antibacterial properties or work as anti-depressants.

Many different essential oils serve the same purpose but are preferred one over the other depending on their aroma and personal preferences. Following is a list of most popular essential oils available and their properties to help you find the right essential oil for your needs:

Basil

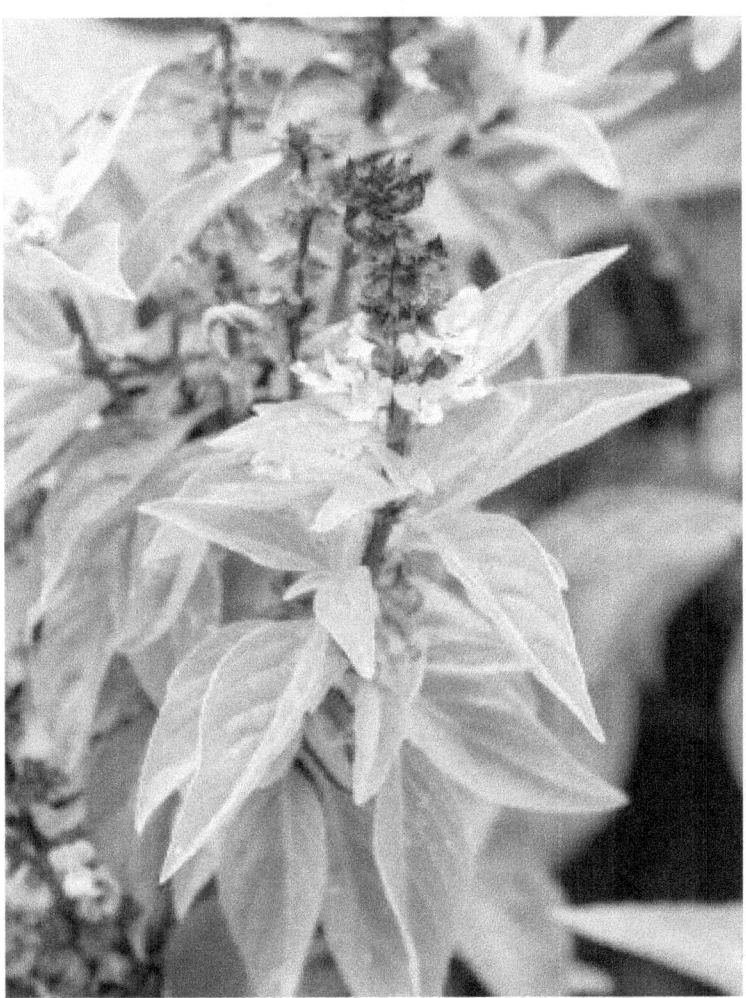

1. It is great for treating ear aches, viral infections, wounds and mental and

   physical fatigue.

2. It stimulates alertness and concentration.

3. It is effective in offering relief from colds, whooping coughs and influenza.

4. It is very beneficial for treating stomach cramps, flatulence, constipation and

   indigestion.

5. It is best paired with lavender, lemon, clove bud, juniper and eucalyptus.

Ylang Ylang

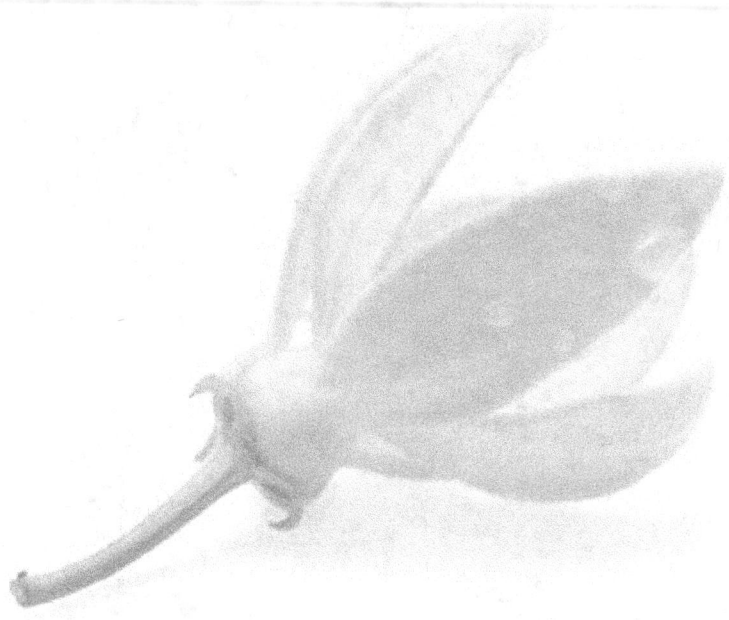

1. It cures internal infections in organs including intestines, colon, stomach and urinary tract.

2. It is a great aphrodisiac and can be used as a natural remedy for loss of libido and frigidity.

3. It has calming properties that are highly effective for anger management. Simply sniff the oil when feeling angry or frustrated and it will calm your nerves.

4. It strengthens the nervous system.

5. It blends well with other essential oils including sandalwood, lavender and

    grapefruits.

Lemongrass

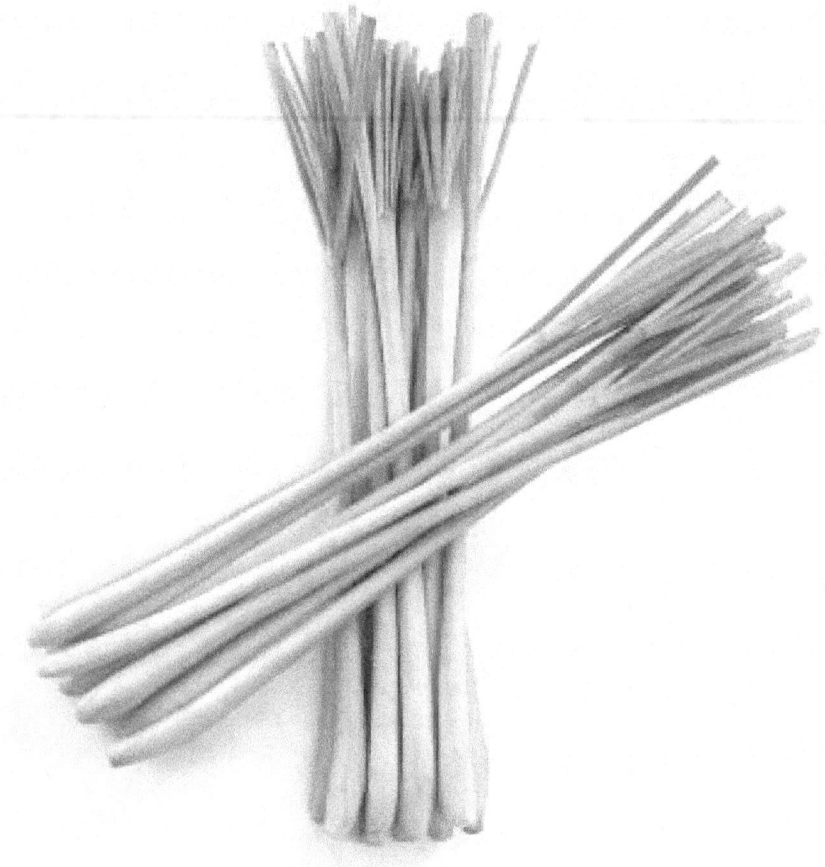

1. Lemongrass strengthens the vascular walls, regulates the parasympathetic

   nervous system and helps in lymphatic system detox.

2. It is very effective for sinus and respiratory conditions.

3. It has anti-inflammatory, antifungal, antibacterial and antiseptic properties.

4. There are over 50 different species of lemongrass, however not all are

   suitable for internal or medicinal use. So make sure you research well before

   making a purchase.

Rose

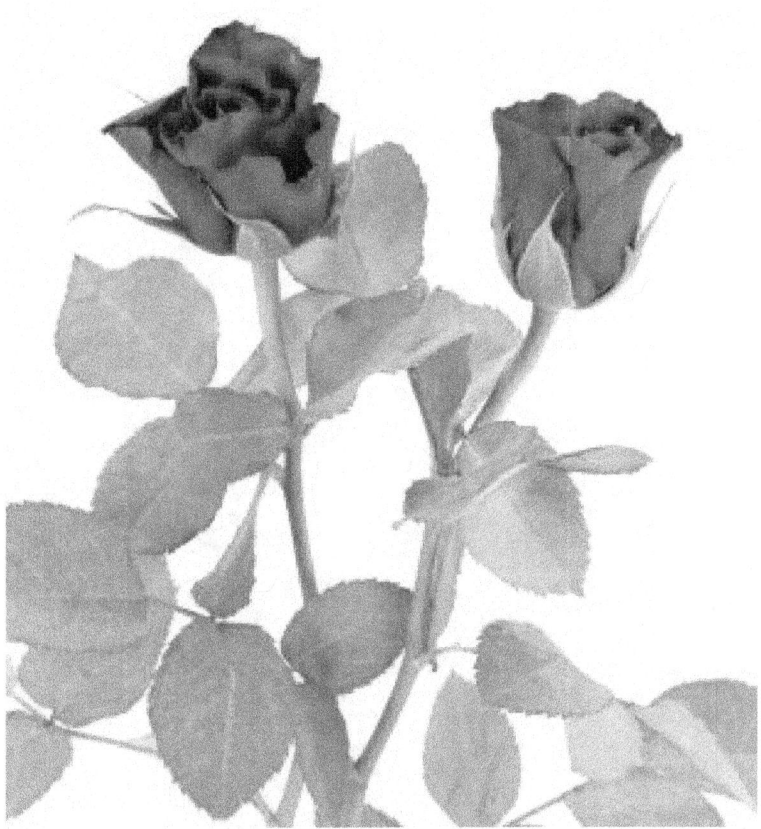

1. Rose is widely known as the ultimate solution for treating depression, grief or

   hysteria. It gives off a light fragrance with great calming properties.

2. Rose is not suitable for pregnant women.

3. Apart from being an effective antidepressant, it also has antiseptic and

   antiviral properties.

4. It has astringent properties that help strengthen gums and hair roots. It

   contracts intestines, blood vessels and muscles.

5. It is highly beneficial for skin. It lifts the skin and gives it a youthful and fresh
   look.

Ginger

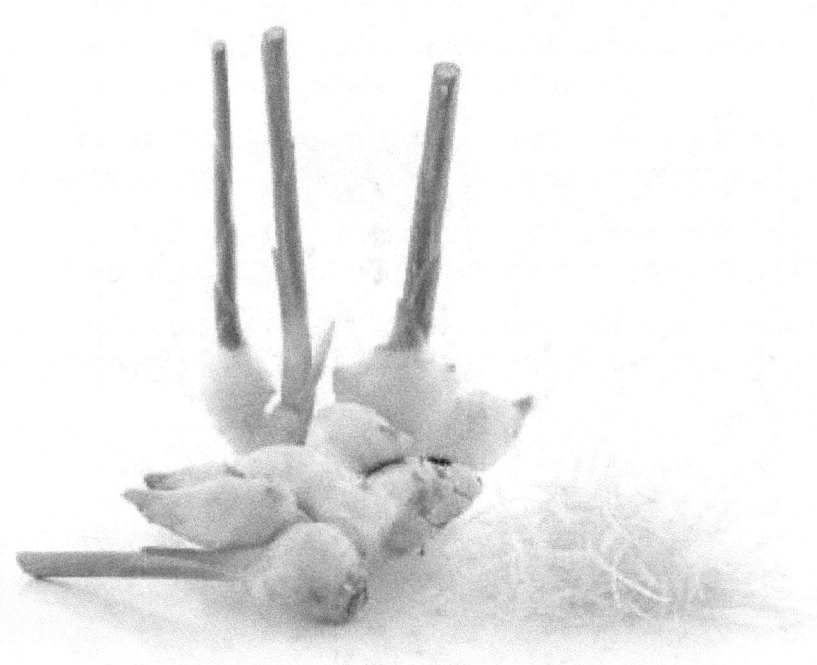

1. Ginger is commonly used to treat nausea and morning sickness. It is suitable

   and very effective for pregnant women.

2. It has detoxifying properties and helps increase blood circulation.

3. It is very useful for those suffering from arthritis.

4. It is best paired with juniper and lemon.

Sandalwood

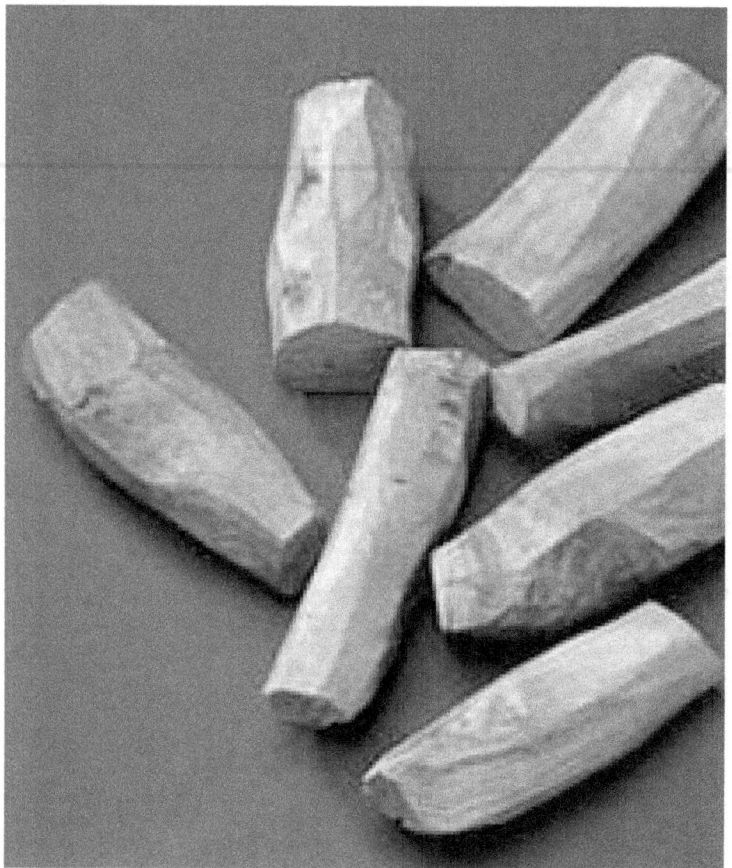

1. Sandalwood has a very aromatic woody smell, making it highly popular with

    men as an aftershave tonic.

2. It dramatically increases the moisture levels in the skin and is widely used as

    a tonic for dehydrated skin.

3. It can also be used to heal sore throats.

Wild Orange

1. Wild orange can help to get an even complexion and reduce wrinkles.

2. It is used to treat mouth ulcers, sedation, bronchitis, heartburn, acid reflux and

   stomachaches among many other ailments.

3. It is effective in lowering high cholesterol level and treating constipation,

   diarrhea, water retention and obesity.

4. It has great anti-depressant properties; making it a great cure for emotional

   strain, anxiety and stress.

Tea Tree

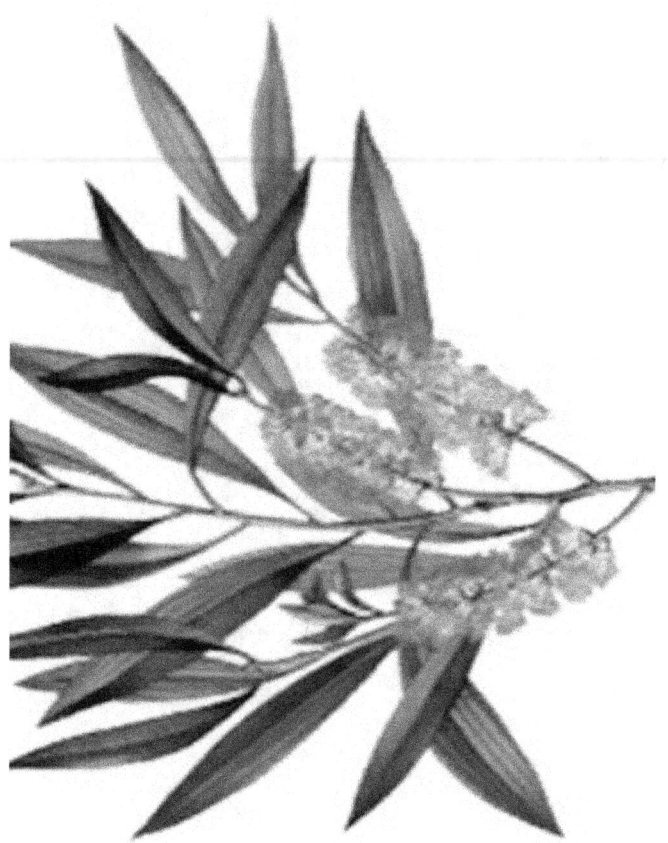

1. It has antifungal properties and is used to treat athlete's foot, fungal infections and nail viruses.

2. It is mostly known as a 'cure all' oil because of its antibacterial and antiviral properties.

Eucalyptus

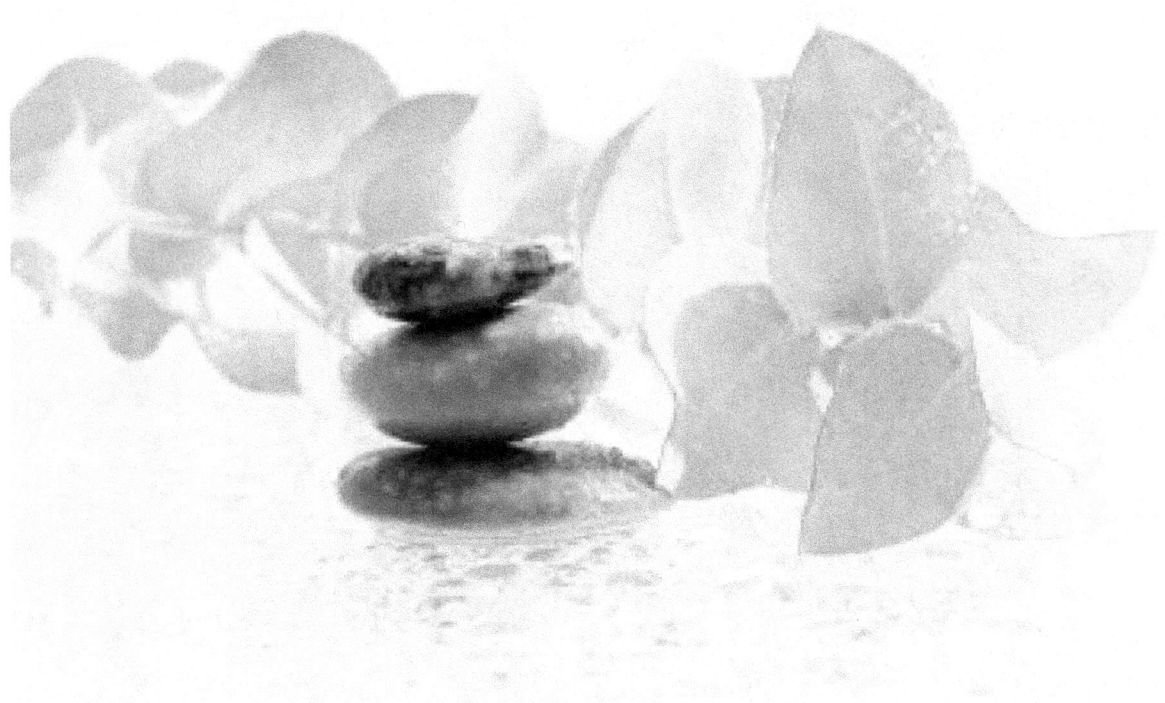

1. Eucalyptus is very effective in relieving muscle and joint pain.

2. It can also be used to treat respiratory problems.

3. Eucalyptus essential oil is not suitable for children.

Chamomile

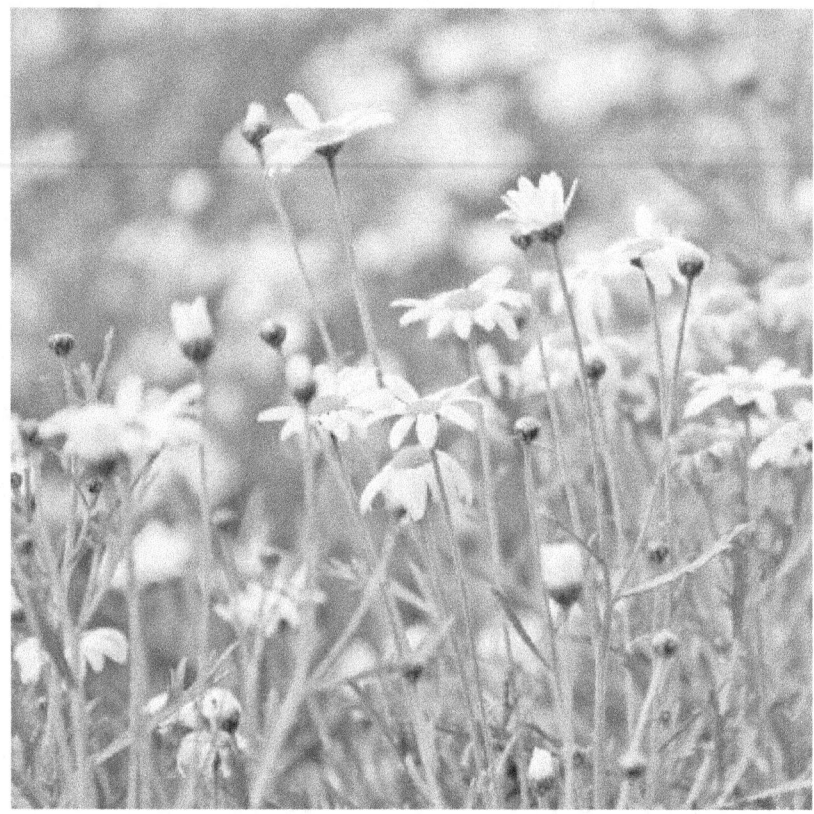

1. Chamomile is effective in calming the nervous system.

2. It helps promote new cell growth.

3. It is very useful in treating acne and dry skin.

4. It can be used to cure inflamed or irritated skin.

Chapter 5 – Storage and Precautions

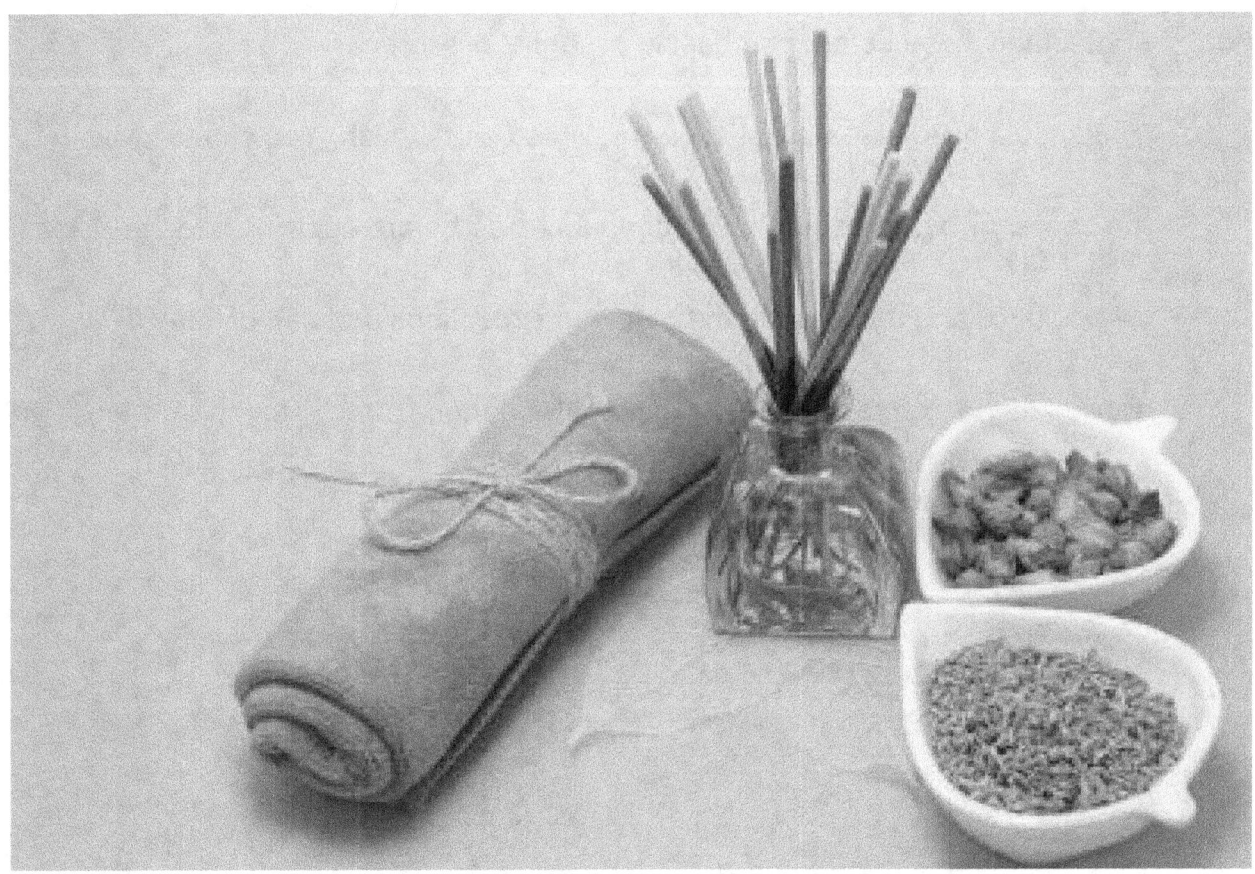

It is imperative that essential oils are used according to instructions to get the best results. Essential oils should almost never be used without carrier oil or undiluted. Essential oils are highly concentrated and if not used carefully can propose health risks. Following are a few precautionary measures you should take when using essential oils:

a) Some essential oils can lead to allergic reactions and irritation in some people. Not all essential oils are suitable for everyone and there are some that should be completely avoided in particular conditions like hypertension, asthma or pregnancy. Some of the potentially dangerous essential oils have been mentioned later in the report, make sure you carefully read and understand those before purchasing essential oils.

b) You should never use essential oils undiluted on the skin. You can mix it with the carrier oil or a cream or lotion of your choice before applying it to the skin. Lavender oil and tea tree are the only true exceptions that can be directly applied to the skin. You should avoid applying these directly to the skin too if you have sensitive skin.

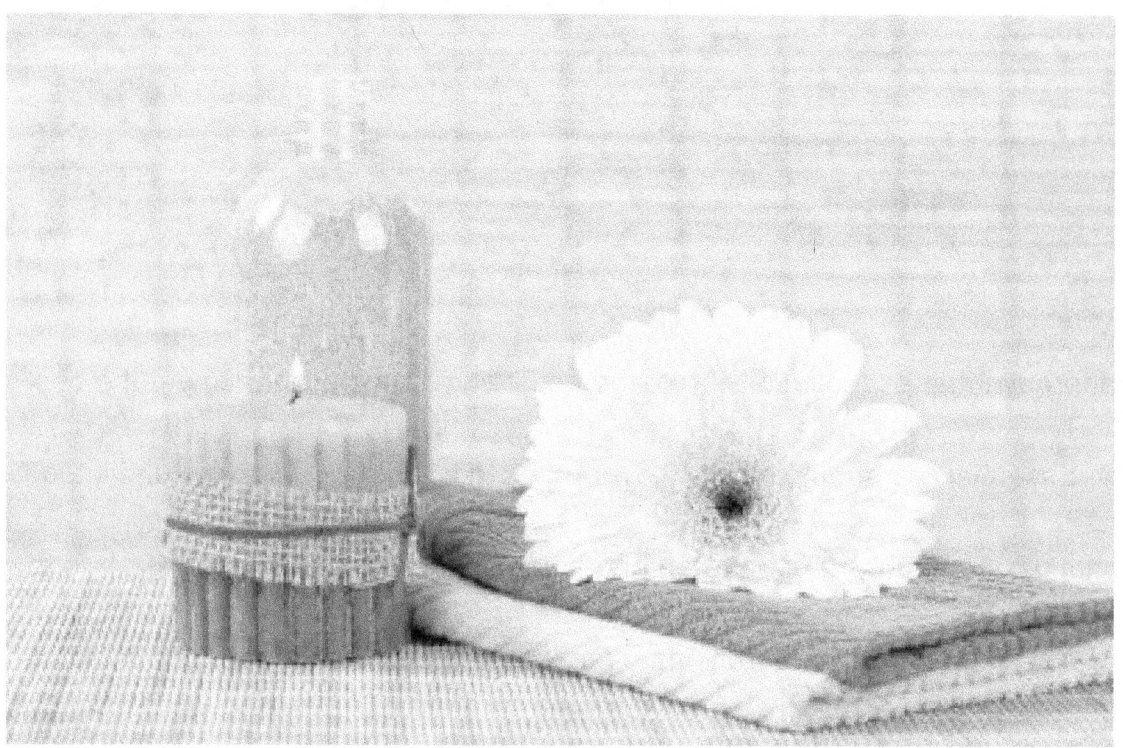

c) Make sure you do a small patch test before applying it to the rest of the body. Seek medical help immediately if you experience itching, burning, redness or irritation.

d) Essential oils are inflammable and should be kept away from any potential fire

hazards.

e) Do not allow children to use essential oils without adult supervision.

f) Make sure you speak to your medical practitioner before using essential oils

for internal use.

Oils You Should Avoid for Various Conditions

Not all essential oils are suitable for everyday use. Some should only be used by a qualified practitioner. Essential oils are highly effective, provided you apply them correctly. Various restrictions like age, skin type and health and medical condition should be considered before using essential oils.

High Blood Pressure

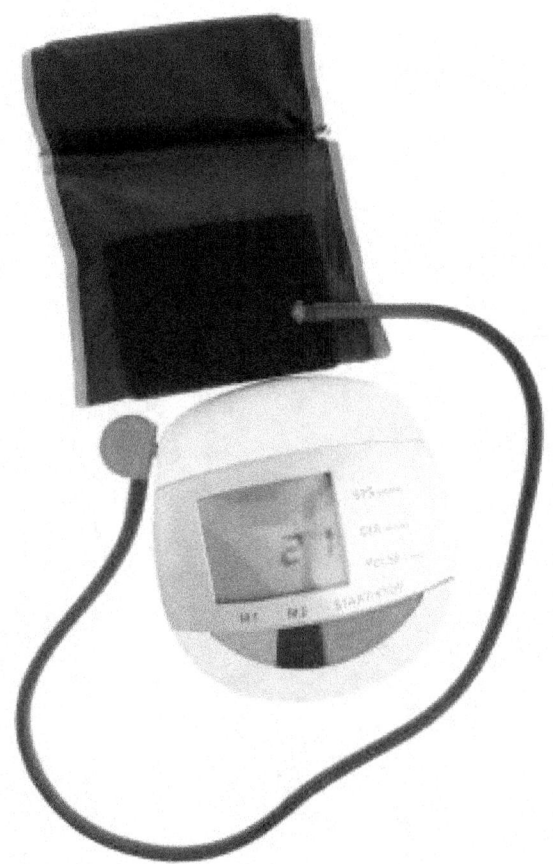

Following are a list of essential oils that people with high blood pressure should avoid because they are stimulating and can further increase the blood pressure:

    i.   Rosemary

    ii.   Sage

   iii.   Thyme

   iv.   Hyssop

Dermal Irritation

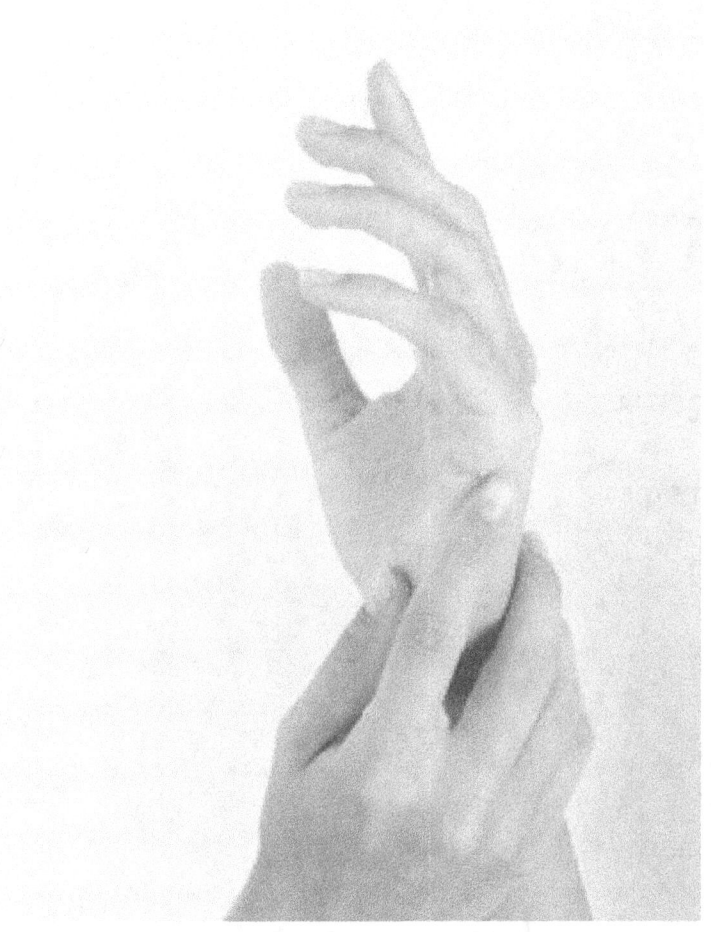

People with sensitive skin should use highly diluted essential oils. If you have

sensitive skin, make sure you use half the strength of all the essential oils when applying. And never use more than three drops when preparing a bath. Limit the overall usage of the following essential oils:

    i.   Aniseed

    ii.   Ajowan

    iii.   Cinnamon

    iv.   Allspice

    v.   Sweet basil

    vi.   Eucalyptus

    vii.   Turmeric

    viii.   Parsley

    ix.   Peppermint

    x.   Lemongrass

Diabetes

    i.   Angelica

    ii.   Rosemary

According to studies, both these oils can increase the blood sugar levels.

Phototoxicity

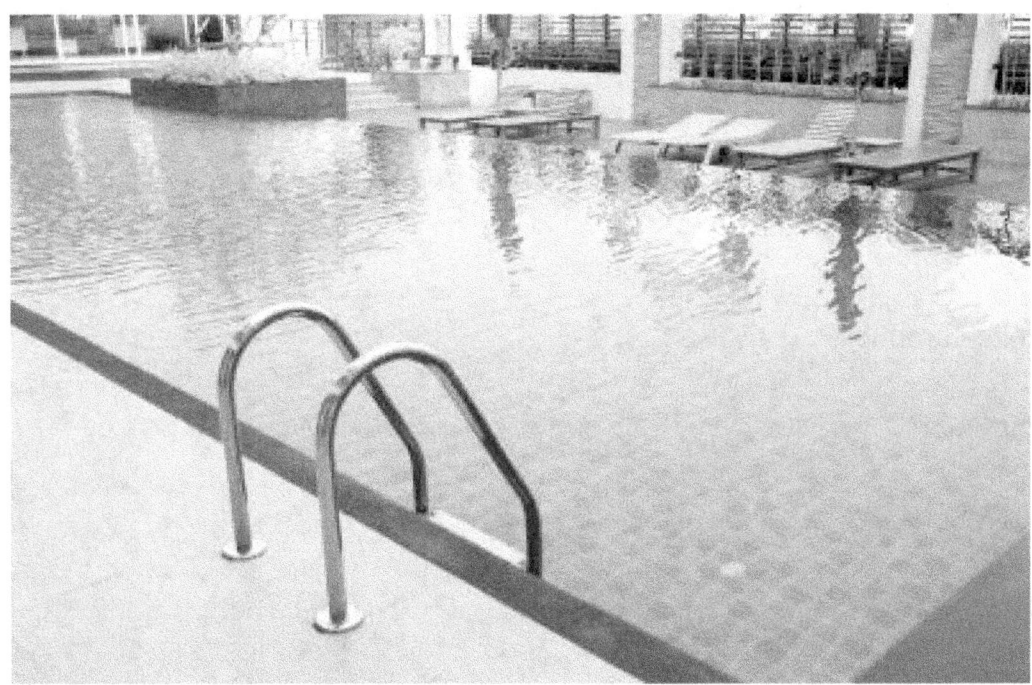

Certain essential oils can cause irritation and skin pigmentation when exposed to direct sunlight after application. Phototoxic essential oils include:

    i.   Bergamot

    ii.   Cumin

    iii.   Ginger

    iv.   Mandarin

    v.   Orange

    vi.   Lime and lemon

    vii.   Angelica root

    viii.   Verbena

Toxicity

Essential oils with high toxicity levels should only be used in moderation. These include:

i.   Exotic basil

ii. White camphor

iii. Cinnamon

iv. Clove bud

v.   Eucalyptus

vi. Sweet fennel

vii. Nutmeg

viii. Turmeric

ix. Turpentine pine

x.   Parsley

Toxicity

Conclusion

Aromatherapy is highly effective and very useful. It greatly helps in increasing the quality of life due to its anti-depressant and natural components. Nature has always provided us with the answers and solutions we are looking for to make our lives easier and more close to our natural being. And aromatherapy makes the best use of what nature has to offer to put our body, mind and soul in sync.

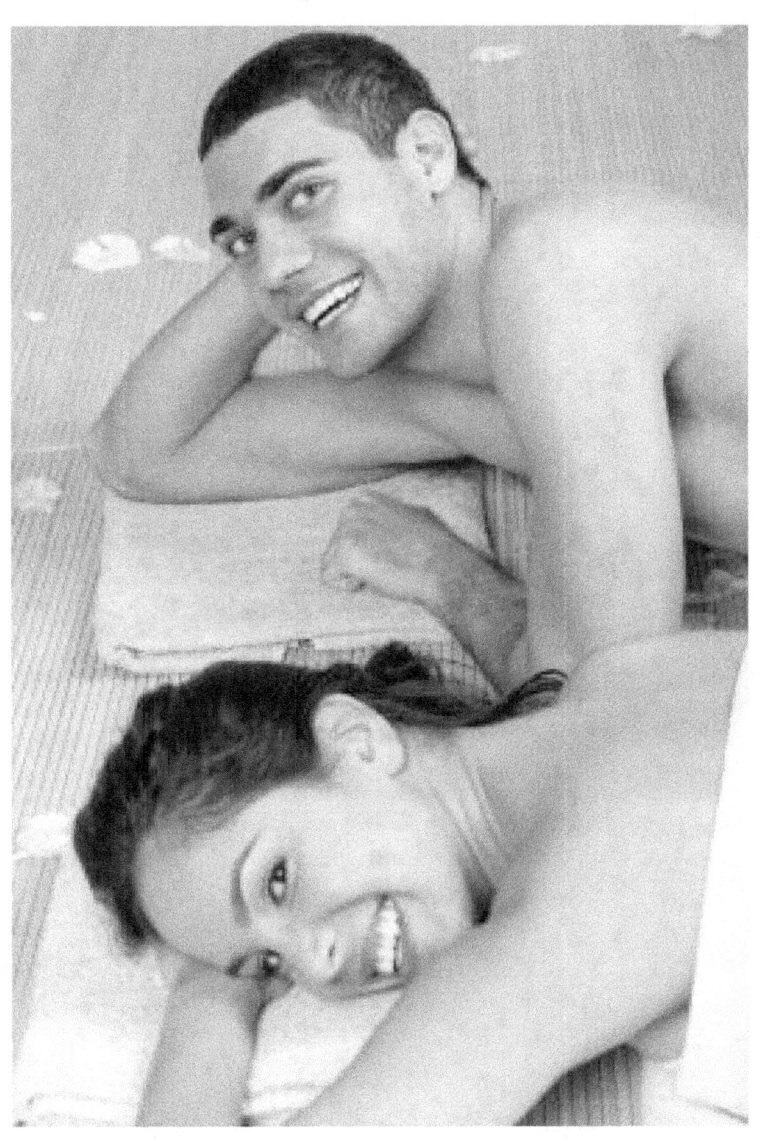

Essential oils today are being used in all parts of the world for various ailments and purposes. Aromatherapy is neither an art or a science, it is just a simple method which when used according to the guidelines can greatly benefit you.

Make sure you purchase undiluted essential oils of high quality without any added 'flavors' or 'scent' for best use. Don't forget to experiment with a number of essential oils to find your personal favorite and let the natural elements take care of the rest!